SEX LORD: A GUIDE TO GRINDING HER LONGER IN BED

DICKSON PETER

Copyright© 2020 Dickson Peter

All Rights Reserved

TABLE OF CONTENT

INTRODUCTION

In this book, we would be looking at the study of the sex organ and control of the sex organ to achieve our goal which is a better and longer sex.

The male sex organ is so full of life and energy and virility, and for quite a long time, it has been an intriguing subject of discussion and a muse for art.

This book would infuse you with a healthy dose of confidence in the life of this interesting sex organ, and if you possess it, you should be proud too. You are about to embark on a journey of blissful pleasures.

CHAPTER 1

PENIS ANATOMY

So for what reasons are we are we looking at the anatomy of the penis? This is because you cannot control what you don't understand. You are going to figure out how to maximize, take care of, and control this organ to the end that you perform better, longer and all the more pleasurably on the bed, wall, kitchen table or in the woods. To accomplish this, you need to understand the components, complexities and scope of this special organ. Therefore, let us get right into it.

The penis is the male sex organ, reaching its full size during puberty. In addition to its sexual function, the penis acts as a channel for urine to leave the body. The penis is made of several parts:

1. Glans (Head) Of The Penis

In uncircumcised men, the glans is covered with pink, clammy tissue called mucosa. Covering the glans is the prepuce. In circumcised men, the prepuce is precisely removed and the mucosa on the glans changes into dry skin. Possibly this is the reason uncircumcised men have greater sensitivity down there, and are bound to get STIs.

2. Corpus Cavernosum

Two segments of tissue running at the edges of the penis. They appear to be flexible, similar to your rubber band. Blood fills this tissue to cause an erection.

3. Corpus Spongiosum

A segment of sponge-like tissue running along the front of the penis and consummating at the glans penis; it loads up with blood during an erection, keeping the urethra - which goes through it - open.

4. The Urethra

You most likely knew about this one in your fundamental science classes. It goes through the corpus spongiosum, directing pee out of the body.

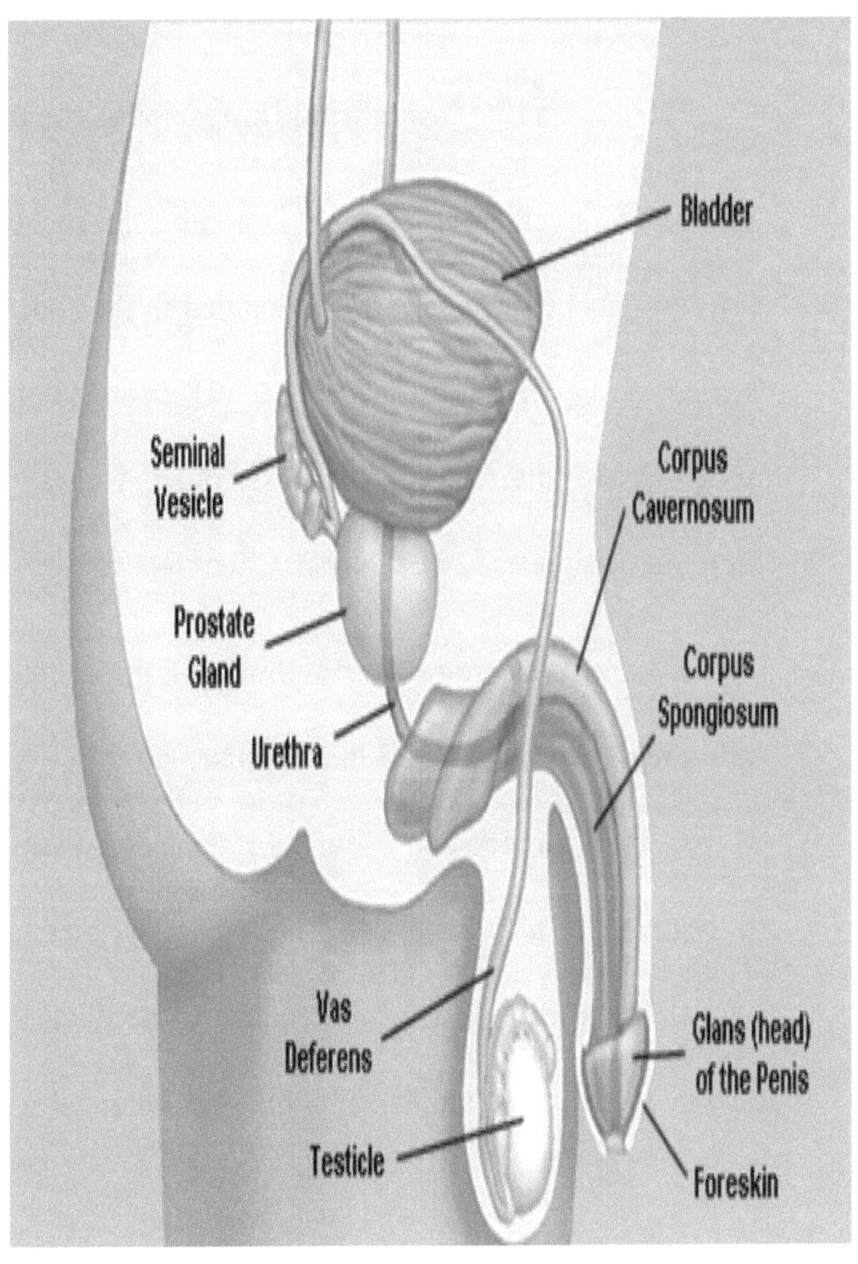
Bladder
Seminal Vesicle
Corpus Cavernosum
Prostate Gland
Corpus Spongiosum
Urethra
Vas Deferens
Glans (head) of the Penis
Testicle
Foreskin

Here are some fascinating things about the penis:

1. The average erect penis is about 5.56 inches (14 cm) long, as per a recent report detailed in the Journal of Sexual Medicine that overviewed 1,661 men. Men in that review had individuals that ran from 1.6 inches (4cm) long to 10.2 inches (26 cm) long. Check your ruler!

Not all erections were made equivalent. The individuals who estimated their penises after oral sex or intercourse brandished bigger penises than the individuals who depended on fantasy alone, the investigation found. And in light of the fact that it decreases blood stream to the penis, smoking can shorten the normal penis by up to 0.4 inches (1 cm), different examinations have found. Indeed, quit that smoking, kid.

2. With regards to penis, size does matter —in any event for certain ladies. Ladies who are more likely to have vaginal orgasms state it is easier to climax with men who have longer penises, as indicated by a recent report distributed in the Journal of Sexual Medicine.

Though it is not clear why this is so, a more extended penis might be better ready to stimulate the vagina and the cervix, study co-writer Stuart Brody, an analyst at the University of the West of Scotland, told Live Science at that point.

In a recent report detailed in the diary Proceedings of the National Academy of Sciences, analysts reported ladies who said the ideal penis size varied with a man's stature, with a bigger organ looking better on taller men.

3. The penis may have been much more alarming in people's developmental past. At a certain point in time, the male penis had spines, however human precursors lost those thorny structures before Neanderthals and present day people separated somewhere in the range of 700,000 years ago, as indicated by a recent report distributed in the diary Nature. That must have really been scary!

4. Regardless of whether men are chaste during the day, their penis is always working out around evening time. Most men have three to five erections per night during

the rapid eye movement (REM) period of rest, regardless of whether they are dreaming about grandmother or Mia Khalifa. This evening time activity clearly keeps the male part fit as a fiddle.

5. Penis anxiety or penis shame is real and normal: In one investigation distributed in September 2013 in the Journal of Sexual Medicine, 30 percent of a sample of British men was very disappointed with their penis size.

The examination found no connection, though, between size anxiety and actual penis size. A few men were so worried about their penis size that they dreaded others would be able to see the size of their organ through their jeans.

If you have this shame or anxiety, not to worry, this booklet would destroy it, giving you a good dose of confidence to go to war (read as bed-matics) with your weaponized organ, and come out the real man, the man whom the woman respects. It doesn't do well for your ego when a woman says you're a one minute man with no atom of respect, does it? We're here for you and that's what this book is for.

In the year 2013, I had the same problem. In fact, the day my first girlfriend left me, she threw insults at me publicly, including the dreaded word, "one-minute man".

No man wants to be called that.

Well, I consider that a compliment because I don't even think I lasted up to a minute in bed. After she left, I was full of defeat and self-esteem issues. I stopped picking up girls, and even developed a hostile attitude towards them.

In the year 2014, I started researching on the ways to last longer in bed. Let me just tell you now that most of the information on the internet regarding this subject are shitty or just plain ridiculous. I was thus faced with the task of trial and error. This journey took me various places, from the shady hotels in Denver to the black neighborhoods in Los Angeles. I tried both the mystic and the medical.

After three years of searching, I was able to separate out the effective methods and techniques from the bullshit, and I would tell you this for free, there is a whole lot of bullshit; from products that don't work or that literally set your penis on fire, to techniques that sound like they originate from the movie, Mad Max. Well, I worked with the effective ones, improved on them and voila, here you have them in this book.

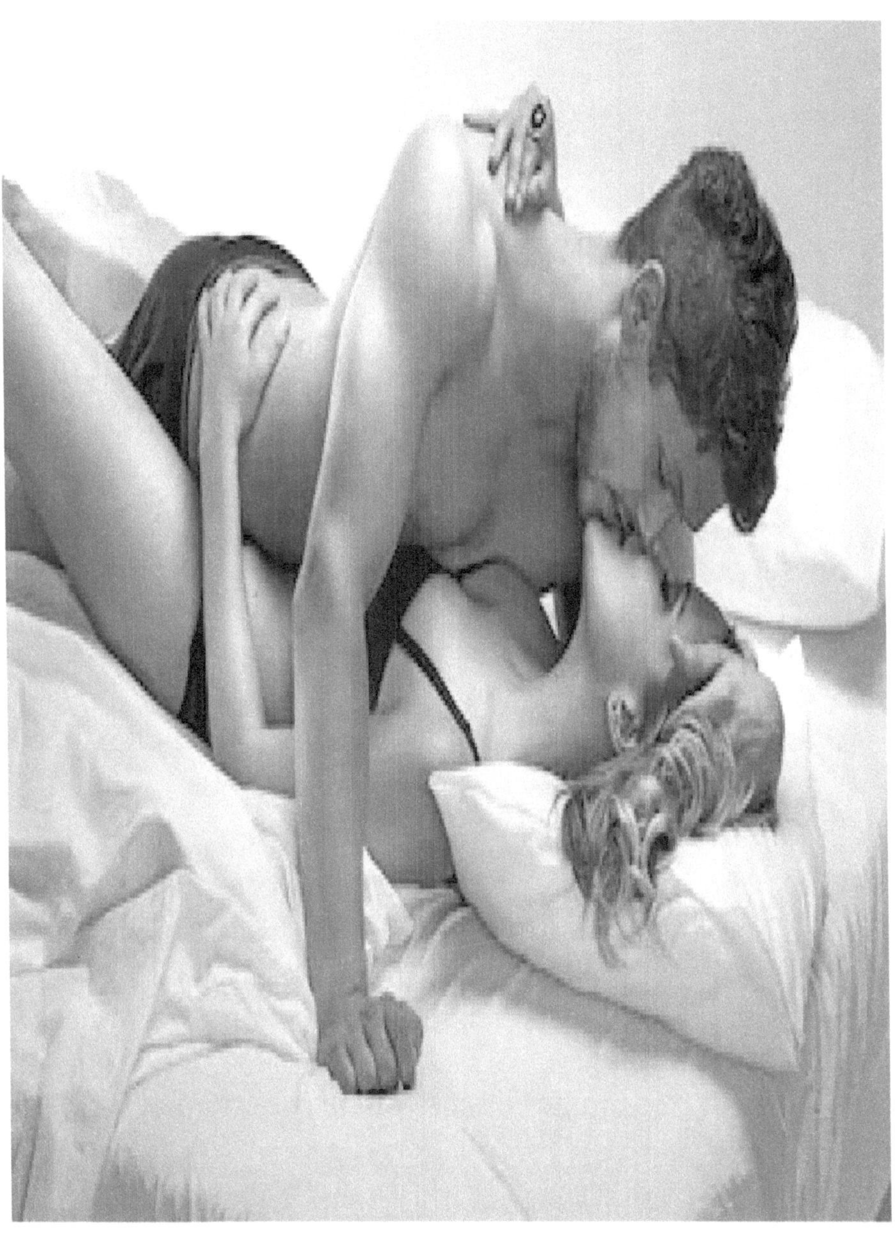

CHAPTER 2

WHAT HAPPENS TO THE MAN DURING SEX

When a man gets aroused, the nerves surrounding his penis become active, making the muscles around the arteries to relax and more blood to flow into the penis. The extra blood makes the penis solid and hard, or erect. This erection contracts the veins so the blood can't leave the penis, allowing the penis to stay erect.

The man will typically insert his penis into the lady's vagina after the above procedures have started. (It is difficult, though not impossible, to insert a flabby penis into a vagina. Essentially, vaginal fluids makes the procedure a lot simpler.)

The erotic joy of sex comes in large part from the movement of the penis (in a thrusting movement) in the vagina. This pleasure builds up until orgasm is reached — though that climax may come at various times for the two partners or maybe just for one partner. Orgasm accompanies increased blood pressure, pulse, and strong contractions in the loins. For men, this is promptly followed by ejaculation.

After a man discharges or if his excitement dulls, detumescence happens, in which the cerebrum sends a signal to permit the blood to leave the erect penis, and it comes back to its flabby state.

THE BASIC SEX POSITIONS AND THEIR CONTRIBUTION TO PREMATURE EJACULATION

At the point when you begin engaging in sexual relations, you get the chance to find that there are a few styles where you last longer and others in which you less. Let's take a look at the two most fundamental positions:

The Missionary Position

The missionary position is close to the male-superior position; that is, the man on top, the woman on the bottom.

My exploration and research too has indicated that if a man is straining his muscles, as he should do to hold himself up during missionary position; it influences his ability to control ejaculation, so this position can worsen issues of premature ejaculation.

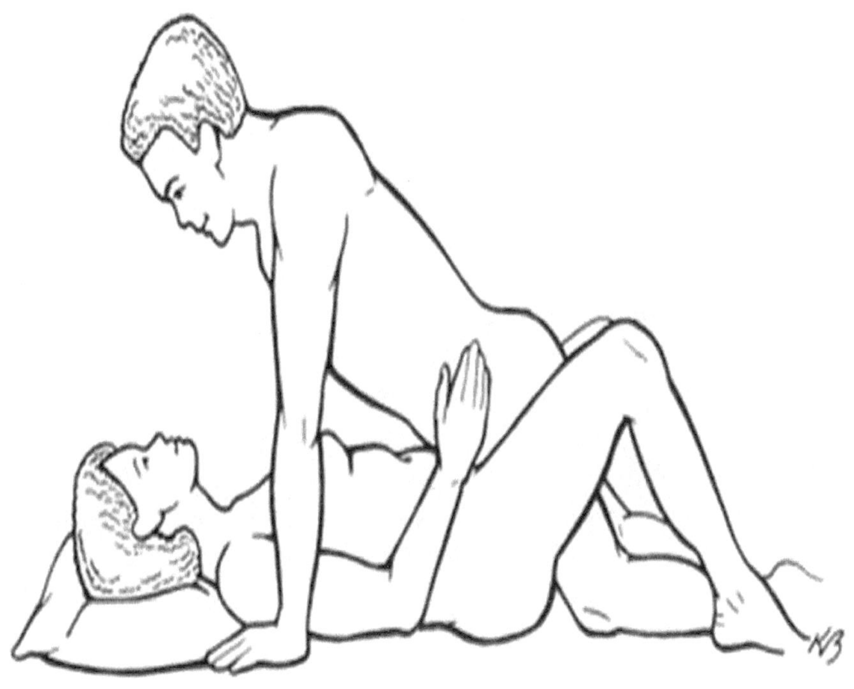

So this position ought not to be your best option, however you can improve it by having the woman lie on a level surface like the kitchen table top while you stand.

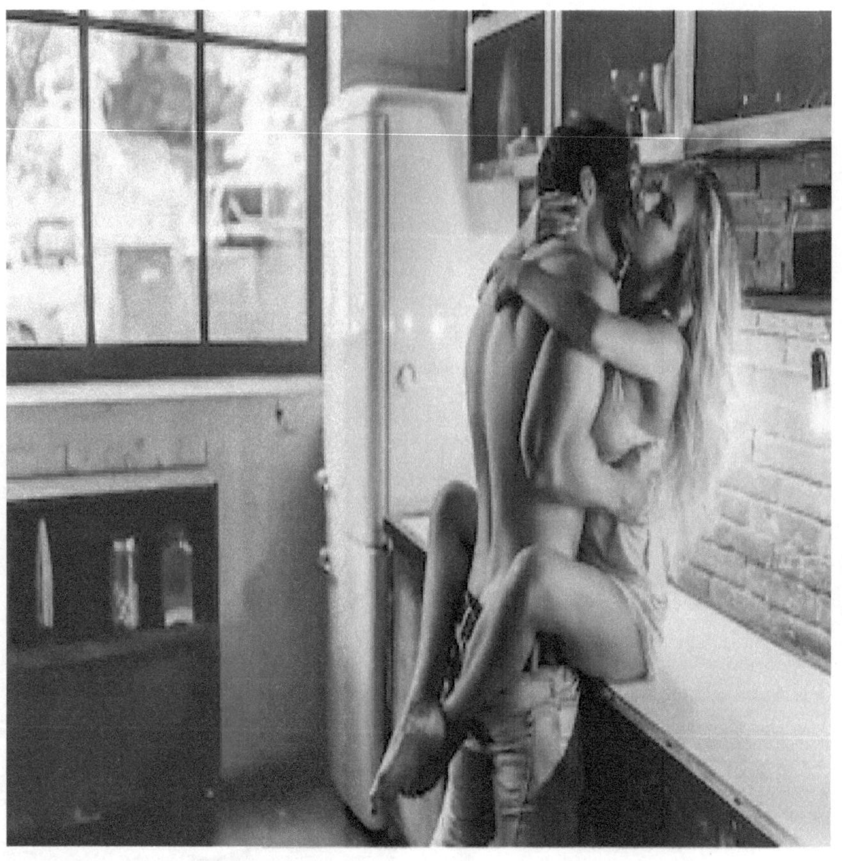

Positioning yourself this way will produce better results, you will last very much longer and have a great pleasurable sex.

The Cow-Girl Position (Lady On Top)

The female-superior position is basically opposite of the missionary position: the lady on top, the man on the bottom. This has become a more common position in the most recent decade or two.

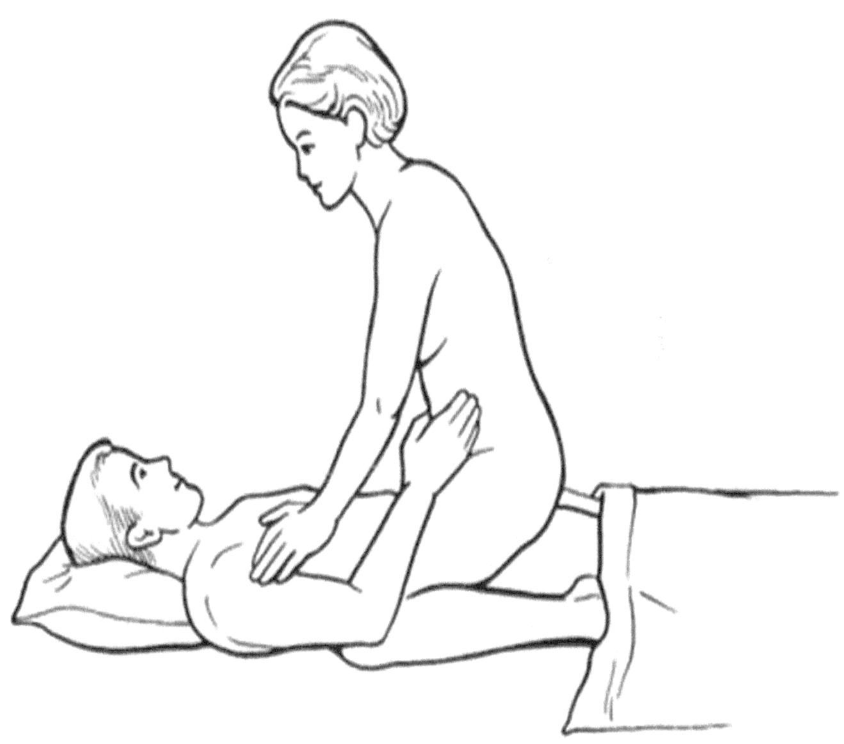

Also, few men have report lasting longer in this position. Nonetheless, the man must have a solid erection for it to work, so it is better in the first part of the day.

You need to explore different styles to discover what works for you. However, subsequent to studying this material and applying it, you would have the capacity to last longer in the different styles that exist.

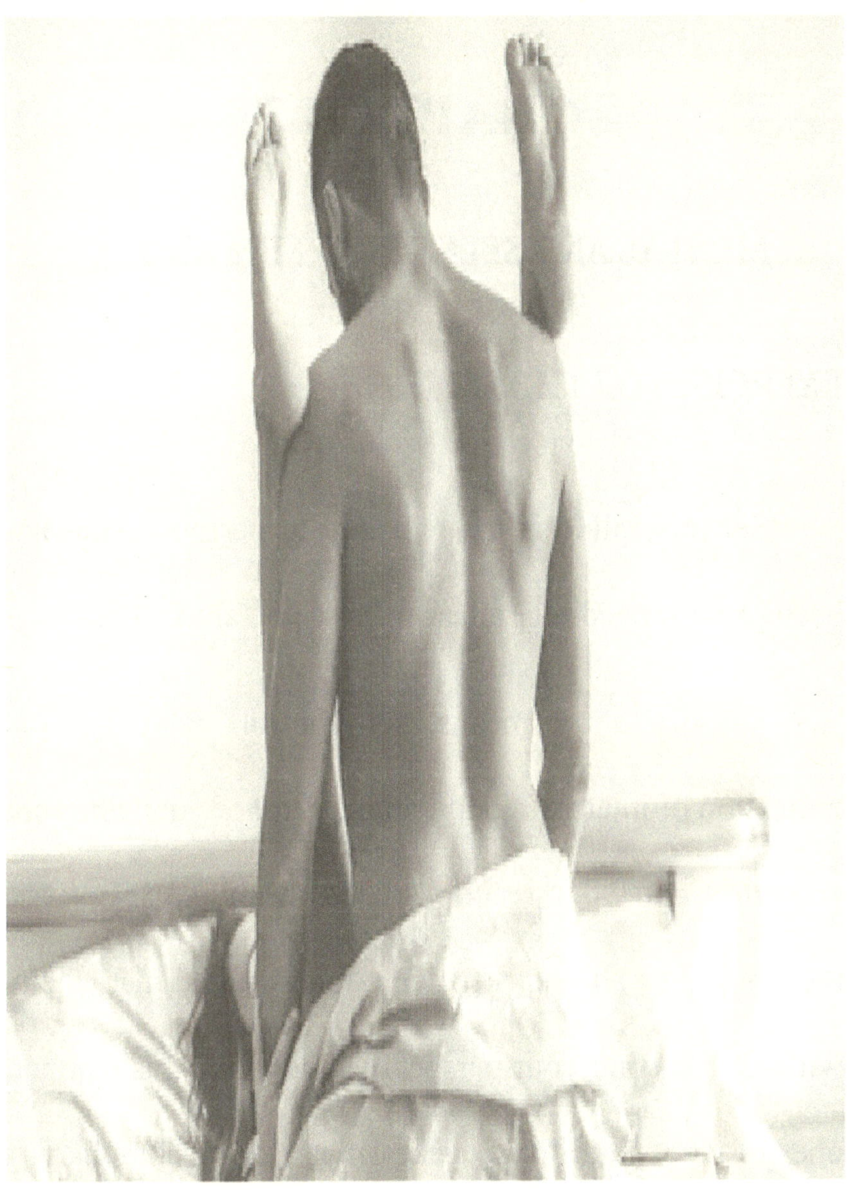

Sex Lord: A Guide To Grinding Her Longer In Bed

CHAPTER 3

MENTAL AND SELF DISCIPLINE AND

EXERCISES OF THE SAME

Self-discipline is the capacity to perform what has been pre-arranged regardless of how you are feeling.

Self-discipline means self-control, which is an indication of internal quality and control of yourself, your activities, and your reactions. Self-discipline gives you the ability to adhere to your choices and finish them, without adjusting your perspective, and is in this manner, one of the significant necessities for accomplishing objectives.

How does self-control come to play in your sexual life?

In the strategies which you would in the end master from this book, you would discover that there are times where you should quit thrusting, and times in which you should continue onward. Without self-control, you would keep thrusting in times when you should stop by reason of the extreme pleaure rocking you. Even your pull-out game is most likely not solid because of absence of self-restraint. You cannot afford to do things dependent on your emotions. This really goes for all parts of life. The man that develops self-control would be good all round, including in bed.

Presently, nobody, I mean completely no one was brought into the world with self-control. Actually childhood is characterized by gross indiscipline. Children do things as a result of how they feel. They want to eat something from the beginning; they want to get it sharply. That is the way life is for them. What I am trying to state was that no one was brought into the world with self-control. It is something you need to develop by practice.

Recall what I said; self-control is following up on an arrangement regardless of how you're feeling. By buying this book, I am assuming that you have made a decision; to last more and better in bed, to be the topic when young ladies congregate and to make them blush when they're examining said topic… or you are a man dedicated to one partner and truly need to do better. To achieve this plan of yours, we have plans and techniques and directives in this book. Would you be able to stick with them, even when you're in the throes of pleasure in between her legs?

Now the way to build self-discipline is to perform daily an action which might not be comfortable in the present but beneficial in the long run e.g running an hour everyday no matter how you feel. But in this book, we'd be focusing on activities that would have a direct impact on your sex life.

PRACTICALS

Endurance masturbation:

Now get naked. Yes.

Rub some lotion or Vaseline on your hands and begin to stroke while mimicking some thrusting movements with your hip. Here is the catch, you must spend nothing less than ten minutes.

You must not cum before then.

How do you do that? Let's assume an imaginary scale to pleasure (you should find out yours practically).

9.5 is the closest point to the so-called "point of no return" when you cannot but cum and 1 is just the beginning moments of arousal. Most people stroke from a point of 1 straight till they nut everywhere. But that is not we are going to do.

Now, stroke yourself to the 4.5 point…then…

Stop stroking (remove your hand bro!).

When you get down to a 3, begin stroking again, to a 6

Stop stroking again till you move down to 4.5 or so

Then begin stroking again till 9.5

Stop till you get down to 3

Then stroke till nuts burst.

At the point when you first begin this activity, it would be a little hard to keep the instruction, "quit stroking". In any case, keep on. Practice till you can last 10 minutes before stroking till finish.

Meditation And Affirmations:

Meditation has been shown to improve self-discipline. Meditation in this context is to empty the mind and focus on the breathing. It is a relaxation technique because as you calm the hyperactive mind, you have a sense of relaxation. Most men who are afflicted with premature ejaculation usually are tense and have thoughts of defeat before and during sex. This sets up a vicious cycle that condition their mind to trigger ejaculation earlier. We'd therefore start from reconditioning the mind with meditation and affirmations. Affirmation is simply to repeat a statement or desire or assertion over and over to yourself. This also reconditions the mind as it changes the way you perceive and view yourself.

How about we get to it

For meditation: get into a relaxed position, preferably the lotus position (have you seen Buddha monks in movies meditating? Yes, that position). Begin to focus on nothing else but on your breathing. Focus on breathing in and out deeply. Do this for about two minutes or so.

Now, see yourself in your mind's eye lasting long in bed. 10 minutes, 20 minutes, you're still thrusting. Imagine the girl's expression of awe, how she's thinking, 'what a man!

Hold this mind picture for as long as you can go. (if you have an erection while doing this, pay it no mind)

Now, after you come out of your reverie, say the following to yourself over and over again. (You can do it in front of a mirror):

I am a strong man

I am the man that lasts 10 minutes in bed

So good am I in bed that girls flock to me

Keep affirming these daily. Affirmations are important to development in all aspects of life including this one. If you can't see yourself lasting long in bed, then you're right, it'd never happen.

The point of these meditations and affirmations is that a very important part of the sexual process is the mind or psychology. If you go into sex with an anxiety or shyness, you are most likely not going to last up to average. The most important sexual organ is the brain, not the penis, so it is important to deal with any anxiety that would prevent you from being at your best during action.

CHAPTER 4

BASIC EXERCISES AND TECHNIQUES

We are first going to consider the basic techniques people use to last longer in bed, before we proceed to the maestro techniques in some detail

Basic Techniques

1. Foreplay

Sex is more than simply penetration. Foreplay can greatly increase the sexual experience in terms of both time and pleasure.

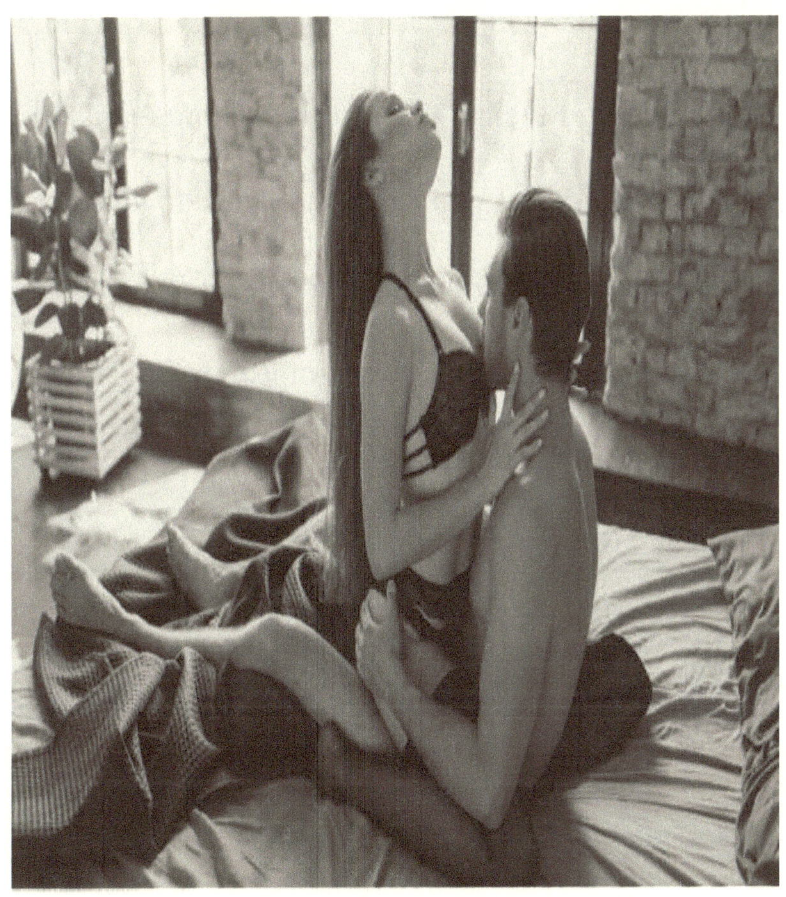

2. Behavioural Techniques

Try the 'squeeze technique', and the stop-start technique.

• Squeeze technique: in this technique, as you near climax, let's say at point 8, you clamp down hard on the tip of your organ with your fingers. To really be good, you really need to know your point 8 or 7, as this doesn't work as much if you are in 9.5.

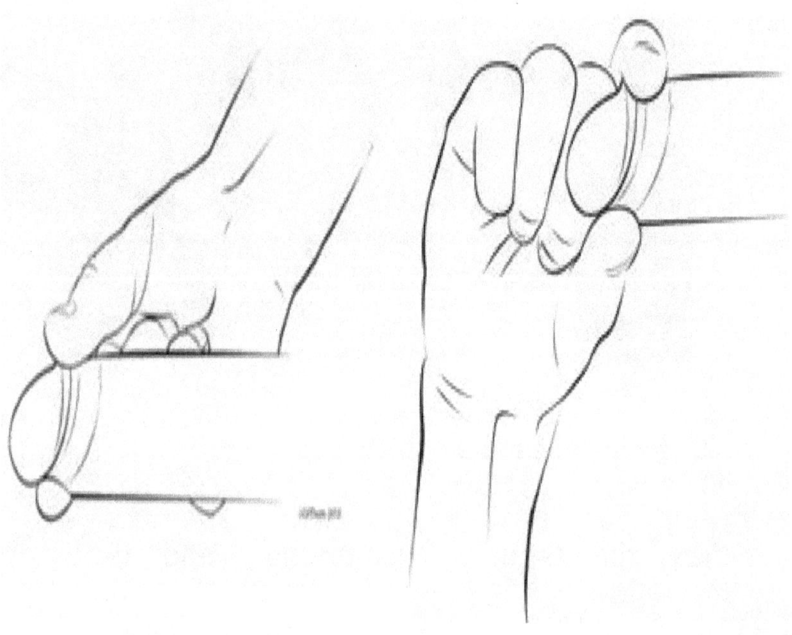

• Stop-start technique: same as above except that in this case, you pull out and rest your organ. You can then continue other foreplay activities while resting it till you probably get to 4.5

3. Mental Distraction

An old classic. During sex focus on your attention on something deeply un-erotic such as multiplication tables. This can reduce the enjoyment of the act itself but is often effective in delaying ejaculation.

4. Slow Down

Generally, the faster the man has sex, the quicker he ejaculates. Rapid, hard thrusts result in a faster climax. A slower, more measured technique means the penis tip is less stimulated and ejaculation delayed. It also allows for greater control over ejaculation.

5. Condoms

Condoms decrease sensitivity and therefore usually increase the time taken to ejaculate. They also have the added bonus of preventing sexually transmitted disease and unwanted pregnancies.

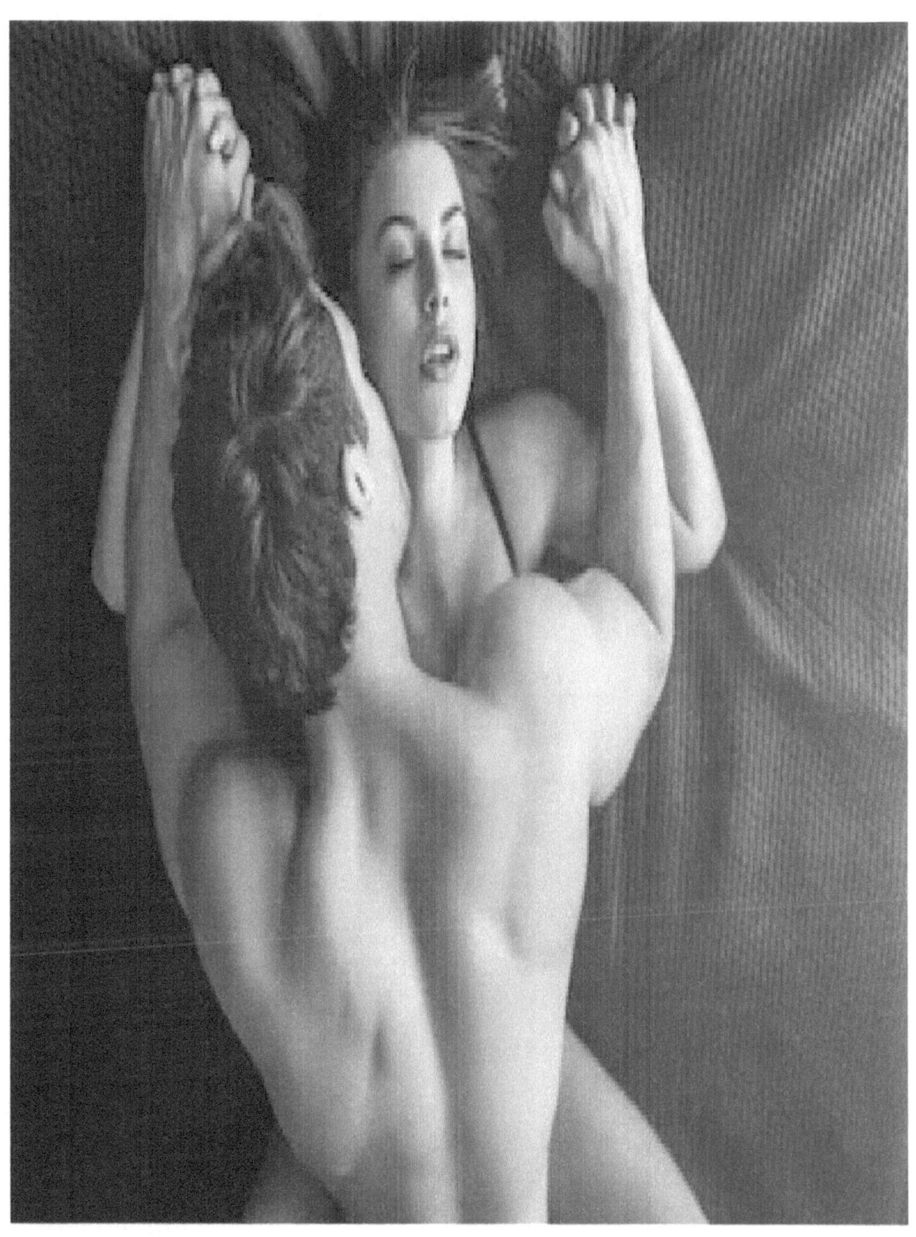

CHAPTER 5

MAESTRO EXERCISES AND TECHNIQUES

The most logical way to control how long you last is to control when you ejaculate. Understand?

And so the way to control when you ejaculate is to strengthen the muscles involved, that is the muscles that control ejaculation.

A powerful way to exercise and strengthen these badass muscles is by kegels and reverse kegels. You can do this exercise less than 3 minutes a day and not only does it help you last longer in bed or in the kitchen, it also can give you more intense and longer-lasting orgasms, and if done correctly and long enough, can get you to the point where you have orgasms without ejaculation.

Sounds powerful right?

Also you can do this exercise anywhere as it doesn't require bending or jumping or even lifting weights with your penis.

So how is this simple exercise done?

First you need to locate your pelvic floor muscle and this is the muscle you will be flexing.

Finding this muscle is by putting a finger on the skin behind your balls but before your anus and flexing that muscle you flex if you were trying to pee.

So with your fingers on the area mentioned imagine you were trying to urinate. Flex that muscle and you should feel movement in that area.

If having trouble go and pee and try to stop yourself.

The Kegel Exercise

This exercise is simply flexing that muscle a number of times for different durations. As that muscle gets stronger you get better in ejaculatory control.

A simple way to do this exercise is this:

1. Flex the muscle hard for 5 seconds un-flex for 2 seconds then repeat for as long as possible.

2. Then flex and un-flex quickly for as long as possible.

3. Flex the muscle hard for 10 seconds, un-flex for 5 seconds then repeat.

The important thing here is not how many times you repeat the exercises daily but how consistent you are in it. You have to be consistent. Consistency always beats intensity.

You can do this exercise 4 times a day if you can, then slow down to once a day for maintenance as the muscle get stronger.

Using This Technique in Bed

To last longer in bed all you need to do is take a few seconds to squeeze that muscle as hard as possible anytime you feel like you are getting too close to orgasm. In the beginning you can let your partner know so they can give you few seconds.

Also before you even get very close to orgasm which we said is a level 9 on the arousal scale remember the techniques we used in our masturbation exercise. To make the movement from a higher level on the scale to a lower level faster, combine the kegel with the TAB technique:

Think: think about something else such as the multiplication tables.

Avoid: avoid the head of your penis instead of stopping entirely.

Breathe: take deep "with your stomach" breaths.

Keep practicing these techniques till they become second nature to your sexual routine.

The Reverse Kegel Exercise

The previous exercise tightens the muscle over and over again to strengthen it. However tightening that muscle can sometimes increase how quickly you get to a level nine as contraction of that muscle is partially responsible for orgasm and consequently, ejaculation in the first place.

Tightening that muscle to the point of exhaustion is how kegels slow you down but this reverse kegel slows you down by relaxing.

When combined together a reverse cowgirl keeps you at the level 4-6 and brings you back down when you climb higher why the normal cake girl saves you at the last minute.

How to do this exercise is to apply internal pressure against those same muscles.

A way to do this is to first push out your ass as if you are going to fart then exhale heavily and try to move that pressure away from your botox into your penis.

This is a more unfamiliar sensation than the kegel so it might take some time to find it. Just keep pushing according to the same timing and variation of the previous exercise we have outlined. **This means:**

1. Push against the reverse muscle for 5 seconds, release for 2 seconds then repeat for as long as possible.

2. Push and un-push quickly for as long as possible.

3. Push hard for 10 seconds, un-push for 5 seconds. Repeat.

As the muscle gets stronger it will get easier to find it and it will feel more natural.

Using This Technique In Bed

During foreplay while receiving oral sex you can apply this pressure to bring yourself down within an accepted level.

During sex, while thrusting, push out with the reverse muscle to stop the over tightening of the pelvic floor muscle and keep yourself at an even level.

This works best while she's on top as it makes it easier to focus your efforts on pushing and since she being on top is a good position as we earlier said, this increases the effectiveness significantly. Don't use your abs to press your hips against her pelvis was as it will be more difficult in that position to press out the pelvic floor muscle. Disengage your abs even as you press your hips against her pelvis while she grinds.

Another thing; TRY NOT TO FART.

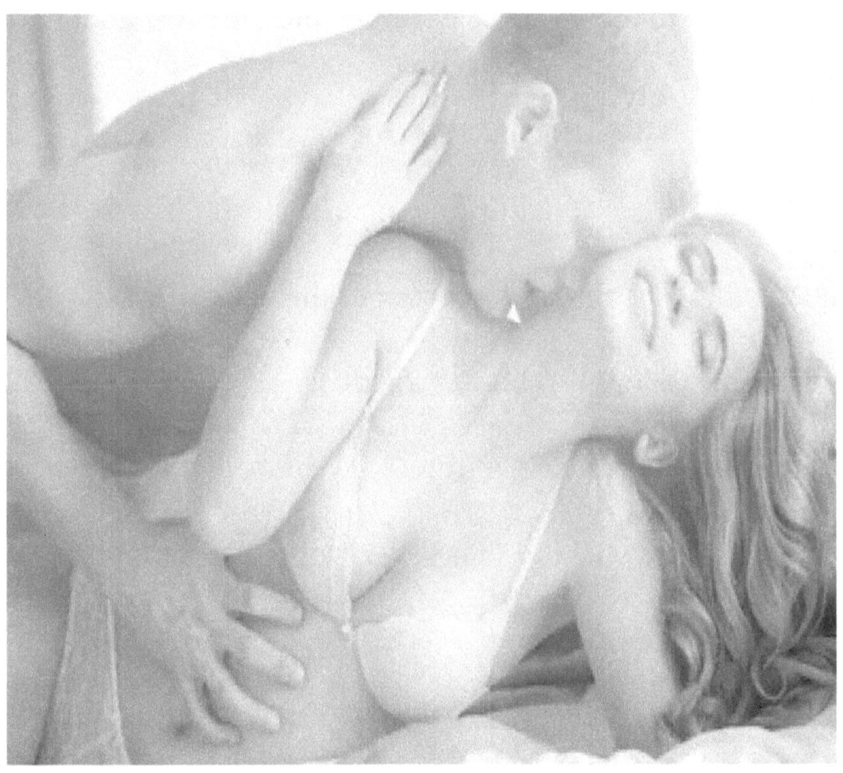

CONCLUSION

Finally, we have looked at ways you can improve the staying power of your manhood and maximize it, ranging from basic and common techniques everyday folks use, to techniques used by the masters and porn stars.

Feel free to tailor the maestro exercises to your needs but let improvement be the goal. Master the guidelines enough to break them in little ways on your journey to becoming a true lord in bed, the tabletop, against the wall, and wherever your tastes might lead you.